Juice Feasting!!!

Juicing in Support of the Health of the Body's Natural Detoxification System

NOREEN KHAN-MAYBERRY, PhD

DEDICATION

For my family and friends throughout the world!

"I'm only aging on Paper!!"

-Dr. Noreen, The Tox Doc

NOTE TO READERS

Juicing is great to supplement any diet! However, you should always consult your physician if you are taking medications or have been diagnosed with a medical condition. An all juice diet is not recommended as a permanent of long-term nutrition plan.

www.DoctorNoreen.com

http://www.youtube.com/user/DoctorNoreen

http://www.facebook.com/DoctorNoreen

@DrNoreen

Disclaimer: Dr. Noreen Khan-Mayberry, aka "Dr. Noreen" does not intend to treat, diagnose or cure. Please consult your personal physician prior to making any dietary changes, especially if you are currently taking medication.

The information and statements contained in this work are the professional opinion of the author and are not endorsed, sponsored or representative of the United States Federal government or any Federal Agency.

Table of Contents

ACKNOWLEDGEMENTS

For those who seek to improve the quality of their lives, I thank you.

INTRODUCTION

Natural Juice: Why juicing is not just a fad!

Many people have asked me why, as a Toxicologist, I am so enthusiastic about juicing. The answer is easy for me. I understand how the body deals with toxic chemicals. Therefore, I want to give my body's detoxification system, the best possible chance of getting rid of those chemicals with the least amount of negative effects. If you have read my book "Talking Toxicology", then you too understand how our body interacts with chemicals. If you have not read this easy to understand guide (I hope that you will), I still applaud you for reading this book so that you too can increase your intake of the most natural form of vitamins and minerals!

Some people think of juicing as a weight loss gimmick. This is not a weight loss guide. However, weight loss is a common effect that accompanies juicing. So while juicing does not guarantee weight loss, it is likely that you will lose some inches/cms or pounds/kilos.

When you juice, you replace some or all of the food in your daily diet with plant based foods. One of the biggest myths is that while you are juicing you are not eating. That is simply untrue. You ARE EATING!! You just are not chewing all of your meals! You will also learn that you are not missing out on proteins and carbohydrates when you juice. People are always asking me, "Dr. Noreen, here are you getting your protein and carbs?" I get them from my juice and you will too. The key is to juice a wide variety of fruits and vegetables to that you can meet all of your body's needs.

Generally speaking people do not ask so many questions when it comes to consuming foods that they know are truly unhealthy and filled with unknown and hard to pronounce chemicals. I wish they did. I would love to see people consult their physician before they start a 30 – 70 year diet that includes fast and processed foods so that they could truly understand the long term effects on their body. Unfortunately, this is not the norm. This being said, please consult your physician prior to starting a plant based diet, particularly if you are routinely taking prescribed medications, over the counter (OTC) drugs and supplements.

I started juicing years ago and recently replaced all of my meals for 30 days with raw, freshly made juices and I documented much of my journey in social media (www.facebook.com/DoctorNoreen). Now just because I juiced for 30 days, does not mean that you should attempt a juice feast without first consulting your personal physician. However, I do not want you to think that you cannot accomplish this and more, because you CAN!!!! I include some of my juice-feast experiences later in this book! I hope that you enjoy reading about my journey. And of course this book has juice recipes!!! Let's start this juice feast!

-Dr. Noreen

1 Juicing & Blending : What's the Difference?

Some people tell me that they are using blenders to juice. Unfortunately, they really are not juicing. If using a blender, you are creating a smoothie or a blend, not a juice. While there are some high water content low fiber juices that can be put into a blender, such as watermelon (red flesh portion), they still have to be strained after blending in order to remove the solid portion of the fruit. Because a juicer is designed to extract the liquid portion from the pulp and a blender is not. So why is this big deal? The major issue with blending versus juicing is that you are not releasing many of the nutrients that are trapped in the plant fiber when you blend with a traditional or microblender. Juicing releases more micronutrients from the plant cell wall than blending will. People often say to me, I am consuming the fiber which is good for me when I drink a smoothie. Yes, fiber is good for you, but the majority is not digested and is essentially there only to push along the solid waste along the digestive tract. Juicing allows you to strip or break down the fiber to release the "good stuff": vitamins, minerals, enzymes, amino acids that may be trapped within the fiber wall (and there is still some fiber content in juice). Blending does not separate these essential micronutrients from the plant fiber; it does liquefy whatever is placed into it by chopping it at a high rate of speed. A much lower amount of juice is extracted from the pulp and you obtain a thick, liquefied soup beverage.

Smoothies and blends are tasty!! But to get the maximum amount of nutrition from your fruits and vegetables you simply must JUICE!! This is why you should not fall for the marketing that says blenders can juice. Blenders can kill many of the beneficial micronutrients by heating and killing them with high power motors. Juicing, if done properly also does not kill those micronutrients by adding heat from a blender's motor. ANY PRODUCT THAT HAS THE WORDS MIX, MIXER, BULLET OR BLENDER IN THE TITLE IS NOT A JUICER!! I cannot stress this enough.

There are so many types of juicing machines and new technology is coming up with new products for juicing. When I first started juicing, I used a centrifugal juicer and I also had a citrus juicer. I now use a low speed masticating juicer. I will provide you with an introduction of the types of juicers now available:

Centrifugal Juicer

This is probably the most popular type of juicer, since it is relatively inexpensive (compared with other juicers). As I stated earlier I used one for years but you lose a lot of your good juice in the pulp in a centrifugal juicer. If you have wet pulp, you have lost juice and money. This type of juicer forces the juiced item through a blade and spins it at high speed to separate the juice from the pulp. The juice ends up in your collection glass or receptacle and the fiber ends up in a separate container.

A centrifugal juicer with a pulp ejector is the same as the centrifugal juicer except that it ejects pulp through a side opening. Many of the most popular centrifugal juicers include the side ejector. Centrifugal juicers are the most popular due to their ease of use and speed. Many do not require fruits or vegetables to be cut into pieces. However, due to the heat that is added by the high speed motor, this type of juice should be consumed quickly, within 10-15 minutes so that the live juice does not oxidize or die into a form that is it not as nutritious (or as tasty). Average prices of centrifugal juicers range from $30 - $250.

Masticating Juicer

A masticating juicer is another high-speed juicer that "chews" or mashes the fruits and vegetables into a fine paste then presses the juice through a screen, such as a stainless steel screen. Many masticating juicers can process foods such as grinding and blending as well. They can be uses to grind nuts, dried fruit, seeds and sprouted grains. They can also process frozen fruits to make ice cream-like dishes. Some masticating juicers feature a hydraulic juice press. The hydraulic press masticating juicers are the highest in price (over $1000) but are also considered the highest in quality.

The low-speed masticating juicers have also gained popularity for their ease of use and the virtual lack of heat that high speed motors introduce. The low speed masticating juicers average around $300-400 in price. I personally use a low speed masticating juicer. The juice does not oxidize as quickly and more of the micronutrients survive within the juice.

Citrus Manual Juicer

Manual juicers are slow turning and use a conical shaped "blade" to press the juice out of the citrus fruits. This juicer is easy to use and makes fresh citrus juice. It does require more manual labor than the centrifugal or masticating juicers, hence the name manual juicer.

Wheatgrass Manual Juicer

The wheatgrass juicer uses a motor that turns a blade slowly within the juicer (such as cast iron). The juice is pressed out of the wheatgrass or leafy green that is feed into the shoot.

Hand Juicing

There are manual hand-juicing kits that come with a grater, grating board and cloth or sprout bag. This method is the most time consuming, but also works when electricity is not available.

Many people have high and low speed juicers for increased versatility. What is so wonderful is that you can shop around for juicers on the internet and a wide variety of stores. I recommend that you choose the juicer that is best for your lifestyle and budget. A juicer should be in every home in my opinion because fresh juice is the best juice!

2 The Body's Detoxification System

So what exactly is your body's detoxification system that I keep referring to? There are multiple organs and systems that are involved in detoxification of foreign toxins (natural chemicals such as viruses, bacterial toxins and molds/mycotoxins) and toxicants (all toxic chemicals including man-made chemicals). Specifically, the major organs that are involved with metabolizing (biotransformation) and elimination of toxic chemicals are the liver, kidneys and small intestine. The liver plays the greatest role in human detoxification. The liver filters blood from the digestive tract before the blood travels to the rest of the body (Talking Toxicology).

There are 3 phases of detoxification. Most toxic chemicals are highly fat soluble – meaning that they dissolve in fat. During phase I chemicals that are absorbed from food in the small intestine into the blood are filtered by the liver and are metabolized or biotransformed into something that is either more or less toxic by the enzymes of the liver. Phase II works to further detoxify chemicals by addition of enzymes in an attempt to make the molecule more water soluble. Phase III is the elimination of toxic chemicals in a liquid or solid form. This is where the kidneys play a role since this set of organs are highly efficient filter of blood for removal of wastes (See Chapter 4 Mechanisms of Toxicity of Talking Toxicology for a more comprehensive explanation).

Toxic chemicals that cannot be detoxified are stored in our fat (adipose) cells. When we start to burn fat, chemicals that were previously stored in those fat cells are freed and get back into circulation through the blood. These freed toxics can also cause symptoms on their way out of the body. This is why when people start to burn fat, especially at a high rate, they may experience a variety of symptoms depending upon what type of toxic chemicals are now circulating in the body. If you experience adverse symptoms, they will likely pass after a few days. However, everyone is different and it is always important to remain in discussion with your medical doctor in order to communicate the types and frequency of your symptoms.

If the body does not have the correct nutritional fuel that it needs to support the body's detoxification process, a number of adverse health effects will occur. Further if damage occurs to the organs of the detoxification system, the body will not perform optimally and may develop disease. If the body's detoxification system is not functioning properly or is overloaded because it cannot detoxify the amount of chemicals that the body is exposed to at a fast enough pace it can reach a point of saturation toxicokinetics. The body will produce a greater number of fat cells to store the excess chemicals. While those chemicals stored in fat may not have an immediate toxic effect, they can cause toxicity over the long term. This is because you have a chronic exposure to low levels of these toxicants that can become immobilized from fat cells and reintroduced into your body's circulation. Excess fat, not only affects body shape, but adversely affects the body's ability to maintain proper health.

While many products offer to "detox" you, most are simply offering you an accelerated elimination of waste products. Don't get me wrong, carrying excess waste products for excessive time periods is not a good thing, but you should work to get your body's detoxification back in shape by supporting it with the right micronutrients such as spinach, grapefruit, ginger, grape seed extract[1], Vitamin C, Zinc, sylmarin (milk thistle)[2], Selenium,   turmeric (curcumin)[3], quercetin[4], tart cherry, alpha lipoic acid[5], l-carnitine[6]. All of

---

[1] Raina et al. 2013, Food Chem, Toxicology
http://www.ncbi.nlm.nih.gov/pubmed/23831192; Khoshbaten et al., 2010
http://www.ncbi.nlm.nih.gov/pmc/articles/PMC3003214/

[2] http://www.cancer.gov/cancertopics/pdq/cam/milkthistle/patient;
Nematbakhsh et al, 2013
http://www.ncbi.nlm.nih.gov/pmc/articles/PMC3634167/

[3] Chin, et al. http://www.ncbi.nlm.nih.gov/pubmed/23931272; Anggakusuma et al., 2013 (Gut) http://www.ncbi.nlm.nih.gov/pubmed/23903236; Guj et al., 2013 http://www.ncbi.nlm.nih.gov/pubmed/23843878

[4] Li et al., 2013 (Human Expl Tox)
http://www.ncbi.nlm.nih.gov/pubmed/23928830; Sangaj et al (2012)
http://www.ncbi.nlm.nih.gov/pubmed/23024108; Liu et al. 2012.
http://www.ncbi.nlm.nih.gov/pubmed/22728154

[5] McMackin CJ, et al. Effect of combined treatment with alpha-Lipoic acid and acetyl-L-carnitine on vascular function and blood pressure in patients with coronary artery disease. Journal of Clin Hypertension (Greenwich). 2007 Apr;9(4):249-55

[6] Acetyl-l-carnitine and Liver Problems Am J Clin Nutr Michele Malaguarnera,

these plant based vitamins, minerals and phytonutrients (nutrients sourced from plants) have been studied extensively and have shown to support not only liver, kidney and digestive health, but neurological health and benefits for multiple biological systems.

Summary

Detoxification should not conjure images of uncontrollable bowel movements and long bathroom breaks! Detoxification should be supported naturally through natural raw juicing or natural supplements that are sourced directly from plant-based foods. Detoxification should not alter your regular life style if you are continually providing this system what it needs!

Marco Vacante, Maria Giordano, Giovanni Pennisi, Rita Bella, Liborio Rampello, Mariano Malaguarnera, Giovanni Li Volti, and Fabio Galvano; Bykov et al., 2003. http://alcalc.oxfordjournals.org/content/38/5/400.full

3 What am I getting out of this juice? Marvelous Micronutrients!!

Micronutrients are just what you think they are – nutrients that the body needs in small or "micro-amounts". Micronutrients include vitamins, minerals, and enzymes – these are critical for the healthy functioning of ALL of the body's systems. They differ from macronutrients such as carbohydrates, protein and fat, which are essential to the body in large or macro amounts. Micronutrients are AMAZING!!

Micronutrients are critical for cellular functions, the healthy functioning of our neurological, digestive, circulatory and natural detoxification systems. And even though we need them in relatively small amounts, these essential nutrients are often what we are lacking in our daily diets. But it is easy to fix this…especially if you juice. Juicing takes massive amounts of fruits and vegetables and extracts the micronutrients into a live form that is readily absorbed by the body. In other words, you don't have to wait for your body to digest or break down the fruits and vegetables for extraction of the micronutrients – your juicer has already done the work for you!! Juicing also does a better job of getting out or extracting more micronutrients per fruit or vegetable than our overworked digestive systems will! And juicing also makes available the micronutrients that tend to remain trapped in the wall of plant fiber cells and lost through regular ingestion of fruits and vegetable. Again, this is maximum bang for your grocery or farming bucks!! There are very few nutrients that are found in natural food sources that will lead to significant toxicity. However, vitamin toxicity is generally only seen by excessive consumption of synthetic vitamin supplements. Supplements that use natural food sources show evidence of toxic effects.

Vitamins

Vitamins were discovered when diseases emerged in certain groups of people that were missing certain types of fresh food in their diets. Scurvy in sailors and pirates is one of the best known examples. This disease which leads to the sea-men losing their teeth, amongst other symptoms, was essentially cured by the addition of citrus fruits into their diets. Research into what "elements" in the foods cured disease led to the ultimate discovery of vitamins. This is when scientists first realized deficiency leads to disease. The term "vitamin" was developed by Kazimierz "Casimir" Funk, a Polish biochemist who, in 1911, isolated a concentrate from rice polishings which remedied nerve damage in pigeons. Funk named the concentrate "vitamine" or "vital amines" since he thought this extract was "vital to life" and he assumed that it was an amine (an organic compound derived from Ammonia). It was proven that the compounds were not amines but the term vitamin stuck from that point on.

Minerals

Plants are designed to ingest and break down minerals, whereas humans are not. Human ingestion of minerals should be from plant-based sources, i.e., food or supplements made from plant-based sources – or progress naturally up the food chain. Minerals are needed to activate enzymes and are therefore essential to all bodily processes. Cellular processes have a chain of events for proper functions – these functions are started by minerals. Many chronic diseases can be traced to a deficiency in minerals. Obtaining readily absorbable minerals through vegetable and fruit juices is most advantageous!

Enzymes

Documenting the history of the first discovery of enzymes is quite confusing as there are many claims of who first discovered these critical catalysts! Enzymes act as the "party starter"! Enzymes break down food into useable forms of energy (think of digestive enzymes in saliva for initial breakdown and in the stomach for breakdown into tiny particles), they speed up biochemical processes in the body, and they convert other micronutrients and macronutrients into other substances! Enzymes are specialized many of them have one function and one function only. They do what they are designed to do and they do it well! Other enzymes are non-specific and can help with multiple cellular processes.

Amino Acids

Amino Acids are the links that make complex chains of proteins. Amino acids are critical to thousands of bodily processes and they must come from food or plant-based sources in order for our body to be able to synthesize them. There are 8 major amino acids which are commonly referred to as essential amino acids, because deficiencies in these amino acids will lead to adverse health symptoms such as premature aging, lowering the ability to detoxify, diminished immunity, and neurological changes such as mental fatigue or inability to concentrate. Essential amino acids can be found in most plant based foods, which is why juicing is such as great source of amino acids!

Summary

Now you know why getting your micronutrients are so critical for not only living a healthy life, but to ensure the quality of our life in the future! Small adjustments, even if you just add 1-2 glasses of fresh raw juice per day into your diet, can help your body function as it is designed to. A great resource for learning how deficiency in vitamins and minerals lead to deficiency is the book "Talking Toxicology", Chapter 8 Nutritional Toxicology. Here you can also find natural food sources of vitamins and minerals.

Don't hesitate...juice in good taste!

4 Juice Transitioning

Juice Transitioning – what, why and how?

What: A juice transition is a phase or time period in which you prepare your body for full juicing prior to all raw juice and also how you prepare to eating regular foods.

Why: Transitioning is important so that you have a better chance of changing from chewing to juice feasting and decrease the chance of intestinal "back-ups" and hopefully minimize adverse symptoms. Transitioning off is vitally important so that you do not shock your system with hard to digest foods too quickly and also to minimize adverse digestive symptoms.

Note that many people never experience adverse symptoms while others may experience severe symptoms when starting a juice feast.

How: You can set your transition time based upon your schedule. I always suggest getting out a calendar to mark your start dates and ensure that you are planning your transition or juice feast at the right time. To transition you will follow a modified diet and introduce juice into all transition weeks. You can change how long or short your transition time is, but if you are a first-timer, I advise using the suggested schedule. Don't forget to consult with your physician if you are on medication regimen.

Phase 1: Transitioning In

Week 1 (Juice + Routine Foods) (or Weeks 1-2)
You will simply be adding 24-36 ozs of fresh raw juice in addition to your regular meals. You may notice that you will not eat as much as the juice is filling. During this week, include a lot of high fiber raw foods with meals such as salads, snacking on apples, celery and carrot sticks. This will facilitate digestion and removal of stored wastes in the digestive tract. Consume <u>at least</u> ten, 8 oz servings of water every day.

Week 2 (Juice + Raw Meals + Routine Foods) (or week 3)
In addition to 24-36 ozs of raw juice, you will be replacing 1-2 meals per day with raw fruits and vegetables (salads are a common choice, but there are many raw vegan food options available). Consume <u>at least</u> ten, 8 oz servings of water every day.

Week 3 (Juice + Raw meals only) (or week 4)

All meals will be raw vegan meals in addition to 24-36 ozs of juice per day! Consume at least ten, 8 oz servings of water every day.

Phase 2: Juice Feasting!

During this phase you will be consuming at least 8-36 oz of juice for every meal or snack time. You can juice for any time period you set. I suggest a minimum of 7 days, but you can start with 5-days, 10-days or 30-days! Consume at least ten, 8 oz servings of water every day.

Phase 3: Transitioning Out - Back to Solid meals

During this phase you are essentially performing the opposite of Phase 1.

Week 1 (Juice + Raw Meals only) (or week 4)

All meals will be raw vegan meals in addition to 24-36 ozs of juice per day! Consume at least ten, 8 oz servings of water every day.

Week 2 (Juice + Raw Meals + Routine Foods)

In addition to 24-36 ozs of raw juice per day, you will be having 1-2 raw vegan meals per day and vegetarian (cooked or raw) meals. Consume at least ten, 8 oz servings of water every day.

Week 3 (Juice + Routine Foods)

You will be consuming 24-36 ozs of fresh raw juice per day. In addition you can now introduce either 1-2 pescetarian (fish or other sea based animal) meals per day into your diet. And your 3rd meal will be vegetarian or raw vegan. During this week, I suggest lots of high fiber snacks such as raw veggies (carrots, celery, and apples). Consume <u>at least</u> ten, 8 oz servings of water every day.

Sample Transition Meals and Snacks

Now that I have summarized transitioning for juice feasting here are some sample meals and snacks!

Juice + Routine Foods

Meals during this week will be comprised of the following formula:

1) 8-24 oz of Raw Juice
2) 4-6 oz of Sea or land-based animal protein
3) ½ cup – 1 cup of carbohydrate
4) Small side salad

Sample Meal 1:

10 oz of Morning Burst Juice (Apple, Cucumber, Strawberries)

4-6 oz of Salmon (steamed or grilled)

½ - 1 cup cooked rice (brown or jasmine)

Small spinach salad (baby spinach leaves, julienne carrots, sliced cucumbers, chopped walnuts, handful of berries) with raspberry vinaigrette dressing.

Sample Meal 2:
12 oz of Dr. Noreen's Green Juice (Kale, ginger, cucumber, cilantro, parsley, spinach, apples)
4-6 oz grilled or steamed chicken breast
½ - 1 cup cooked rice (brown or jasmine)
Small mixed greens salad (mixed leafy greens, slivers of almonds, julienne carrots, sliced cucumbers, sliced radishes, mandarin orange slices) with strawberry vinaigrette dressing

Sample Meal 3:
12 oz of Dr. Noreen's Green Juice (Kale, ginger, cucumber, cilantro, parsley, spinach, apples)
4-6 oz of Grilled Steak
½ - 1 cup of cooked pasta (any type) or 3-4 small red potatoes (roasted with olive oil)
Grilled vegetables (zucchini, asparagus or eggplant)
Small cup of diced tomato, cucumber and onion salad (seasoned with salt and pepper) with vinaigrette dressing

Sample Meal 4:
12 oz of Apple Berry Refresher Juice (Apples, Cucumber, Blueberries)

Grilled Portobello Mushroom Cap

½ - ¼ cup of pasta or zucchini pasta

Grilled asparagus

Small kale salad (kale, cherry or sliced tomatoes, dried 2 tsp cranberries, 1 tsp sunflower seeds, sliced strawberries, dash salt and pepper, splash lime or lemon juice. Optional parmesan cheese).

Juice + Raw Meals + Routine Foods

During this week you can use meal from the "Juice + Routine Meals" week formula.

This week's Raw Meal formula is:
1) Large raw main course
2) Side salad or trail mix
3) 12-24 oz of raw juice

Note: Depending upon where you live there more raw-vegan restaurants for lunch and/or dinner. Check the internet for locations near you!

Sample Raw Meal 1:

18 oz of Dr. Noreen's Green Juice (Kale, ginger, cucumber, cilantro, parsley, spinach, apples)

1 cup of fruit salad (chopped strawberries, blackberries and raspberries)

Raw Oatmeal:
- 1 cup Raw Oatmeal
- 2 tsp chia seeds
- Handful blueberries (or raspberries)
- 2 medjool dates chopped
- ¼ cup chopped walnuts (or almonds)
- ¾ cup raw almond milk (or any soy or nut milk) or water

Drizzle of Raw Agave Syrup or Raw Honey

Combine raw oatmeal, chia seeds and milk. Let sit for 2 minutes Add chopped dates and berries. Drizzle raw agave on top. Optional – 1 tsp of raw sugar or stevia to taste.

Sample Raw Meal 2:

18 oz of Apple Berry Refresher Juice (Apples, Cucumber, Blueberries)

1 ½ cups of Trail Mix (raw cashews, pistachios and raw almonds, dried cranberries)

Large shredded cabbage salad:
- 2 cups of shredded red and green cabbage;
- 1 ½ cup thinly sliced or chopped apples,
- ¼ cup chopped walnuts,
- ¼ cup dried cranberries,
- ¼ cup raisins.

Dressing:
- ½ tsp minced garlic,
- ½ tsp minced ginger,
- ¼ tsp sea salt,
- ¼ tsp black pepper,

- 2 tsp rice vinegar,
- 3 tsp apple cider vinegar,
- 1 tbl of olive oil,
- 1 tsp brown mustard.
- 3 tsp agave syrup

Combine in blender or food processor.

Sample Raw Meal 3:

18 oz of Sweet Candy Juice (Apples, oranges, strawberries)

Almond Date Mix: 1/2 cup of raw almonds and 4 chopped medjool dates

Raw Veggie wrap:

1 large Swiss chard or collard leaf – trim/remove stem by placing leaf flat with stem side up. Cut stem closely along the edge with knife, leaving a relatively flat leaf.

Dressing:
- 1/2 tsp flax seed,
- 1 tsp lemon juice,
- 2 tsps olive oil,
- 1 tsp of sesame seeds,
- 1 pinch of sea salt,
- dash of black pepper
- 1 piece of garlic.

Directions: Combine dressing ingredients in food processor and spread mixture all over the leaf. Next Stack on top of leaf: julienned or grated vegetables (cucumber, carrots, bell pepper), alfalfa or bean sprouts, thinly sliced avocado, sliced red onions, small sliced tomato, ¼ cup pitted olives, few cilantro leaves.

Roll tightly.

Sample Raw Meal 4:

18 oz of Dr. Noreen's Green Juice (Kale, ginger, cucumber, cilantro, parsley, spinach, apples)

1 cup of fruit salad (chopped strawberries, blueberries, blackberries and raspberries) with sliced almonds

Raw California Roll:

2 Nori sheets, ½ avocado sliced into strips, ¼ cup grated carrot, ¼ seeded cucumber cut into strips, 2 cups of alfalfa sprouts, ¼ bell pepper seeded and cut into flat strips) layer ingredients on Nori sheet, roll into tight roll with bamboo sushi mat. Seal edge with water. Dip in Nama Shoyu (raw soy sauce) and miso – optional.

SNACKS!!!

Tip: It is best to pre-package snacks in small reusable containers!

Trail Mix:
- dried cherries,
- dried cranberries,
- chopped dates,
- cashews (raw, unsalted)
- almonds (raw, unsalted)

- walnuts (raw, unsalted)
- pistachios (raw, unsalted)

Power Berry Mix:

1 cup each of

blueberries,

raspberries,

blackberries

Raw grab and go's: ½ to 1 cup of ANY of the following:

Baby carrots

Celery

Raw almonds

Raw walnuts

Radishes

Fresh Fruit (Any kind)

Dried/dehydrated fruit

Other snack ideas:

Kale chips

Smoothies

Hummus

Granola

Layer raw salad (fruit or veggie) ingredients in a mason jar for an easy to take and beautiful snack.

Summary

There are so many ways to transition into and out of full juice feasting!! You can mix and match with what works for you. If you are a big salad eater, this is a great option for the working person as salads are served at most places. The internet is also a great source for vegan, vegetarian and pescetarian food ideas! Have fun trying new foods!

5 What's in this fruit? What's in this veggie?

A 2008 study published in *Biomedical Environmental Science* provided evidence that kale juice can reduce the risk of coronary artery disease when consumed on a regular basis (Kim et al).[7] This is just one example of the benefits of juicing your greens. And there is mounting evidence that supports the health benefits from consumption of fruit and vegetable based juices that are published in peer-reviewed journals around the world.

But you may wonder what types of micronutrients are in the fruits and vegetables that you consume. As a toxicologist, I most often get asked about organic versus non-organic fruits and vegetables. In regards to juicing, I suggest organic and or locally grown fruits and vegetables. The point of

---

[7] Kim et al. Kale juice improves coronary artery disease risk factors in hypercholesterolemic men. Biomed Environ Sci. 2008 Apr;21(2):91-7. doi: 10.1016/S0895-3988(08)60012-4.

juicing is to support your body's natural detoxification system, therefore you should reduce the amount of chemicals that you reintroduce in your juice. However, if you cannot access or afford organic, you still should juice as raw juicing is a marked improvement over the average diet.

And of course, there is the debate about genetically modified organism or GMOs. A review published in the open access journal *Entropy* provided evidence that glycophosphate the main ingredient in a globally popular herbicide. Glycophosphate residues are found in many foods and it is known to inhibit cytochrome P450 (CYP P450), the main enzymes used by the liver for phase I detoxification. The article goes on to further show evidence that the inhibition of CYP P450 enzymes leads to the decrease in production of amino acids of the gut and impairment of the transport of serum sulfate. The article goes on to argue that the typical Western Diet can lead to chronic diseases such as gastrointestinal disorders, obesity, diabetes, heart disease, depression, autism, infertility, cancer and Alzheimer's disease.

Every day, I read mounting evidence regarding the long term toxic effects caused by GMOs. Many countries have banned the sale of GMO containing foods (including produce). In the US, GMO foods are sold routinely and they are not readily identifiable, since this is not written on the food labels. Hopefully, in the future, labeling will no longer be an issue so that consumers can make informed decisions.

So let's get to the heart of this chapter and that is identifying the types of nutrients that are found in your fruits and vegetables. This quick guide is a tool to help you sort out all of the "good stuff" within your produce!

Vitamin A - Retinol

Sources: Broccoli, Carrot, Dark Leafy Greens, Green Peas, Kale, Mango, Papaya, Pumpkin, Peach, Red Bell Pepper, Spinach, Tomato

Benefits: maintains specialized tissue health such as the retina; aids in normal development of teeth, skeletal and muscle tissue; promotes skin cell growth and healthy skin and mucous membranes.

Note: There are 2 types of vitamin A preformed and pro-vitamin A. Provitamin-A is found in plant based foods, while preformed is found in animal products, including dairy. One of the most common types of Provitamin-A is beta carotene. Generally speaking, the more intense the color of a fruit or vegetable, the higher the beta-carotene content.

Vitamin B – 1 Thiamine

Sources: Green Peas, Spinach, Tomato, Watermelon

Benefits: good for correcting digestive problems such as diarrhea, poor appetite or ulcerative colitis. Boosts immunity, lowers brain inflammation of peripheral nerves associated with pregnancy, stress reduction – adaptogenic properties (helps you adapt to stressful situations). Supports ocular (eye) tissue health. Slows kidney damage progression in those with type 2 diabetes.

Vitamin B – 2 Riboflavin

Sources: Broccoli, Bell Peppers, Kale Spinach

Benefits: promotes healthy reproduction, maintains specialized ocular (eye) tissue health; prevention of migraine headaches, helps boost athletic performance, slows cellular aging, skin development and function, development of the lining of the digestive tract and blood cells. Aids in the production of glutathione, which reduced the amount of free radicals in the blood. Works with other B-Vitamins to metabolize fats, carbohydrates and proteins to provide energy for the body. Prevents hypersensitivity to light. Used to prevent migraine headaches and cataract formation in the eyes.

Vitamin B – 3 Niacin

Sources: Broccoli, Kale

Benefits: antioxidant, blood sugar control, detoxification support – metabolism of chemicals, production of adrenal hormones, production of stomach acid, production of gonadotropin – sex hormones. Lowers bad cholesterol levels by increasing good cholesterol. Supports brain health, healthy skin and hair.

Note: Niacin and Niacinamide are 2 forms of Vitamin B-3, also known as nicotinic acid. Niacinamide is made in the body by the conversion of niacin to niacinamide.

Vitamin B – 6 Pyridoxine

Sources: Avocado, Banana, Green Peas, Spinach, Tomato, Watermelon

Note: Pyridoxine, Pyridoxamine, and Pyridoxal are different forms of Vitamin B-6. Pyridoxine is most commonly found in foods.

Benefits: maintains neurological health, blood health and skin health; maintains blood sugar levels, breaks down proteins in food. NIH[8] states that Vitamin B-6 may alleviate upset stomach and nausea during pregnancy; it may reduce premenstrual syndrome and may reduce depression in children with low levels of serotonin.

---

[8] National Institutes of Health. "Pyridoxine (Vitamin B6): MedlinePlus Supplements". August 2011 .
http://www.nlm.nih.gov/medlineplus/druginfo/natural/934.html; National Institutes of Health. "Vitamin B6: MedlinePlus Medical Encyclopedia". August 2011. http://www.nlm.nih.gov/medlineplus/ency/article/002402.htm.

Vitamin B – 9 Folate, Folic Acid, Folacin

Sources: Broccoli, Green Peas, Kale, Leafy Greens, Spinach, Tomato, Watermelon

Note: Folate, Folic Acid and Folacin are different forms of Vitamin B9. Folate covers all 3 forms of Vitamin B9.

Benefits: maintains blood health, neurological health, prevents birth defects, supports healthy fetus, and may prevent osteoporosis, anti-cancer activity for cervical cancer. Releases serotonin – anti-depressant activity.

Vitamin C – Ascorbic Acid

Sources: Broccoli, Bell Peppers, Citrus Fruits, Kiwi, Mango, Strawberries, Snow Peas

Benefits: immune system health, skin health, bone health, and dental health, cardiovascular health. Loaded with antioxidants, anti-cancer and anti-stroke properties. Promotes cellular healing and has adaptogenic properties (aids the body in adapting to stressful situations). Binds and removes heavy metal toxicants, supports good bacteria formation in the gut, destroys bacterial and viral toxins.

Note: most people, especially children are deficient in Vitamin C, which is mainly found in fruits and vegetables. This is why juicing is especially good for getting enough Vitamin C for your body. Supplementing with Vitamin C/ascorbic acid sourced from natural plant based food sources is also beneficial.

Vitamin E – Alpha Tocopherol

Sources: Avocado, Broccoli, Collard Greens, Green Peas, Mustard Greens, Kale, Kiwi, Papaya, Red Bell Pepper, Spinach, Swiss Chard, Tomato

Benefits: highest in antioxidant activity of all vitamins. Critical for specialized tissue health of brain (neurological system) and gut-brain (enteric nervous system). Prevents break-down of red blood cells.

Note: Alpha Tocopherol is the most active form of Vitamin E in the body. Other types are beta -, gamma- and delta-tocopherol and alpha-, beta-, gamma- and delta-Tocotrienol.

Calcium

Sources: Broccoli, Cabbage, Collard Greens, Green Leafy Vegetables, Kale, Mustard Greens, Parsley, Turnip Greens

Benefits: maintains specialized tissue health of the bone and teeth. Needed by children to achieve full growth potential. Scientific evidence suggests that calcium plays a role in preventing cancer, diabetes, regulating cardiac (heart) muscle contraction, blood clotting.

Note: Children, adolescents and American adults are at risk for calcium deficiencies. Juicing is an easy way to correct this deficiency. Utilizing a natural food-sourced supplement is also recommended.

Chromium

Sources: Apple, Banana, Garlic, Grapes, Orange

Benefits: maintains optimal blood sugar levels by enhancing the action of insulin, energy conversion of fats, carbohydrates and proteins, lowers bad cholesterol, slows calcium loss, beneficial for ocular (eye) health. Prevention of coronary artery disease.

Note: Trivalent (3+) chromium is biologically active and available in food. Hexavalent (6+) chromium is highly toxic and is a product of industrial processes.

Cobalt
(main constituent of Vitamin B12/ Cobalamin)

Sources: Beet Greens, Cabbage, Kelp, Spinach, Watercress

Benefits: maintains specialized tissue health of the bone and teeth. Regulation of cardiac (heart) muscle contraction, blood clotting. Production of red blood cells (erythropoiesis).

Copper

Sources: Avocado, Beet Roots, Bell Peppers, Broccoli, Carrot, Dandelion Leaves, Grape, Green Leafy Vegetables, Kale, Orange, Tomato

Benefits: Essential for adequate use of Iron by the body. Is a part of many enzymes and proteins essential for dealing with Iron. May contribute to lowering cholesterol.

Fluorine

Sources: Apple, Seaweed

Benefits: Supports healthy bones, increases bone density, immune support, strengthens teeth, and reduces tooth decay.

Note: Fluorine is a highly toxic gas, this is different from the element found in trace amounts in food.

Iodine

Sources: Asparagus, Seaweed, Turnip Greens

Benefits: maintains health of the specialized thyroid glands. Supports proper development and metabolism, efficient use of calories, skin, hair and dental health, reproductive health.

Iron

Sources: Avocado, Bell Pepper, Broccoli, Kale, Leafy Greens, Parsley, Peach, Pears, Tomato, Pumpkin

Benefits: essential for proper growth and development. Essential for blood formation of hemoglobin (the main carrier of oxygen in the blood). Supports immunity, aids with insomnia, regulates body temperature (maintains homeostasis). Essential for brain health, muscle health and function.

Magnesium

Sources: Bell Peppers, Broccoli, Kale, Dark Leafy Greens, Garlic, Peach, Peas, Tomato

Benefits: maintains blood pressure, critical in maintaining cardiac rhythm supports bone tissue and dental strength, aids in relief of menopausal and premenstrual symptoms, minimizes risk of premature labor, boosts the bioavailability of Vitamin B-6. Relieves constricted airways of the lung, prevents constipation, osteoarthritis, migraines, kidney and gallbladder stone formation. Aids in absorption of Calcium by the body.

Manganese

Sources: Avocado, Bell Peppers, Bilberry, Blackberry, Blueberry, Broccoli, Carrot, Ginger, Grapevine, Kale, Leafy Greens, Peas, Pineapple, Red Raspberry Leaves, Spinach, Tomato

Benefits: essential in many biochemical processes in the body including utilizing and metabolizing cholesterol, carbohydrates and proteins. Contributes to bone tissue and connective tissue formation. Aids in Calcium absorption and blood sugar regulation. Aids in the production of blood clotting factors and sex hormones.[9]

Molybdenum

Sources: Leafy Greens, Peas

Benefits: Essential enzyme co-factor. Aids in the metabolism of carbohydrates and fats. Facilitates in amino acid breakdown. Aids in energy production, function of the nervous system. Possible anti-cancer properties. May prevent erectile dysfunction. Detoxification support - aids in processing of waste by the kidneys. Suggested that since molybdenum depletes copper in the body, which is necessary for blood vessel production, that in theory, new tissue including cancerous tumors will not grow – much more data is needed to support this claim. Excess molybdenum can lead to anemia.

Potassium

Sources: Apricot, Avocado, Banana, Bell Peppers, Broccoli, Chard, Citrus, Garlic, Grapefruit, Guava, Kale, Leafy Greens, Squash, Tomato

Benefits: Critical for heart beat; maintains cardiac pumping of blood throughout the body. Potassium

---

[9] Manganese. University of Maryland Medical Center.
http://umm.edu/health/medical/altmed/supplement/manganese#ixzz2fesdCDwP

triggers the squeezing of the heart. Potassium can aid in correcting blood pressure disease. Some suggest that potassium also helps lower bad cholesterol. Also critical for kidney function. Deficiency in potassium is associated with the risk of high blood pressure, heart disease, stroke, arthritis, cancer, digestive disorders, and infertility.

Selenium

Sources: Avocado, Bell Peppers, Broccoli, Cabbage, Celery, Cucumbers, Garlic, Hibiscus, Kale, Leafy Greens, Swiss Chard

Benefits: plays a key role in metabolism. Antioxidant, anti-cancer, anti-bacterial, anti-viral, promotes cellular health. Regenerates Vitamins C & E. Critical for reproduction, thyroid hormone metabolism, DNA synthesis, and protection from oxidative damage and infection.

Note: People with H.I.V. and Chron's disease tend to have low selenium levels. Selenium exists in two forms Selenium organic (selenomethionine and selenocysteine) and inorganic (selenate and selenite). Both forms are found in our diets as they are absorbed by plants grown in soil.

Silicon

Sources: Alfalfa, Bell Peppers, Leafy Greens, Horsetail Grass

Benefits: bone and collagen formation.

Sulfur

Sources: Brussels Sprouts, Cabbage, Turnips

Benefits: joint health, anti-inflammatory, essential for glutathione, the top antioxidant for liver health, to function (natural detoxification support). Improves the body's ability to make its own antioxidants.

Zinc

Sources: Bell Peppers, Bilberry, Broccoli, Buchu Leaves, Kale, Leafy Greens, Tomato

Benefits: maintains specialized tissue health of the eye, boost immunity – aids in white blood cell function, anti-parasitic. Improves taste and smell senses. Vital for healthy sperm – protects reproductive cell DNA and prevents breakdown. Works with Vitamin B-6 to ensure brain function.

Summary

So you wanted the evidence as to why plant based foods really are good for you. Now you have it!!! Carry this book forward...but do not lend it to a friend because you will never get it back!

6 Juice Recipes!!

Let's get to it!! Juice Recipes Galore!!
Note: Fist = handful or fistful. Yield will vary depending upon juicer.

Dr. Noreen's Green Juice

Drink it every day!!

3-4 leaves of Kale

¼ - ½ inch of Ginger root (rhizome)

1 large Cucumber

Small fist of Cilantro

Small fist of Parsley

1 - 2 fists of Spinach

4 Apples (sweet variety)

Starter Juice

2 medium Apples

2-3 medium Carrots

1 Cucumber

4 large Strawberries

Handful of seedless Grapes (red, white or both)

1/4 inch Ginger root (rhizome)

Morning Burst Juice

2 Apples

1 medium to large Cucumber

6-8 Strawberries

Apple Berry Refresher Juice

3 Apples,

½ large Cucumber

1 fistful of Blueberries

Pina-lotta Juice

½ Pineapple

1 cup Coconut water or Milk

Sweet Candy Juice

2 Apples

2 Oranges (rind removed)

8 Strawberries

Lighten Up!

2 stalks of Celery

2 Carrots

2 Apples

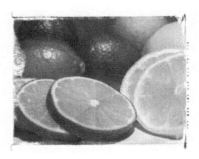

Lemon-Lime Love Juice!!

2 Limes (rind removed)

2 Lemons (rind removed)

½ fist of Parsley

½ fist of Cilantro

4 Strawberries

Add freshly crushed Mint Leaves to juice

Need some Heat!

½ - 1 inch Ginger root (rhizome)

¼ cup Radishes

1 medium Cucumber

1 large Apple (sweet variety)

1- 2 leaves of kale

1 large orange

<u>Simple and Effective</u>

1 – 2 large Cucumbers

2 Green Apples

<u>Mean Greens Juice</u>

3 – 4 leaves of Kale

1 Broccoli floret head with long stem

1 fist of Spinach

½ fist of Parsley

½ fist of Cilantro

4 Green Apples

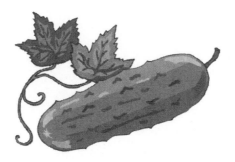

Make your own 8!

2 – 3 Roma Tomatoes

1 – 2 Beet Roots

2 Stalks of Celery

½ fist of Watercress Leaves with stems

½ fist of Parsley

4 leaves Romaine Lettuce

3 Carrots

1 fist of Spinach

Melon Melody

½ of a small seedless or seeded watermelon

½ Cantaloupe (seeds removed)

½ Honeydew (seeds removed)

Note: Juice flesh and rind of the watermelon only.

Do not juice rind of honeydew or cantaloupe.

Purple Paradise

10 large seedless Black Grapes

¼ Purple Cabbage

1 medium Cucumber

6 – 8 Blackberries

A Pear of Kiwi

2 Pears

2 Kiwis (skin on okay)

1 Apple

4-5 large Strawberries

Add freshly crushed Mint Leaves to juice

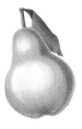

Collard Me Crazy!

3 Collard Green Leaves

3 Mustard Green Leaves

3 Turnip Green Leaves

3 Kale Leaves

1 large Cucumber

2 Carrots

3 large Apples

Beet me Up!!

2 Beet roots

2 Kale leaves

1 Broccoli Floret with long stem

3 Carrots

1 large Cucumber

1 large fist of Spinach

Berry me Happy!!

4 – 6 large Strawberries

½ cup Blueberries

6 – 8 Blackberries

2 red Apples

Zu-Juice

2 medium Zucchini

½ Bell Pepper (any color)

2 Celery stalks

3 large Apples

1 medium Cucumber

1 carrot

¼ - ½ inch of Ginger Root (rhizome)

Evening Energy Fruit juice

20 Red and 20 Black seedless Grapes

1 Green Apple

½ Cucumber

¼ Ginger

6 Strawberries

Super Power Juice!

20 red seedless Grapes

4 leaves of Kale

1 inch Ginger root (rhizome)

2 fist size bunches of Spinach

Fist size bunch of Cilantro

Fist size bunch Parsley

2 Carrots

1 Cucumber

<u>Purple Power Juice</u>

2 leaves of Swiss chard

Small bunch of Green Grapes

2 leaves Purple Kale

1 Cucumber

1 Orange

4 Strawberries

1 Pear

1 Kiwi

2 Red and 2 Green Apples

1 fist of Cilantro

20 Blueberries

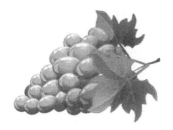

Lovely Green Juice

4 leaves of Kale

2 fists of Spinach

1 Cucumber

4 small Apples

Fist of Parsley

Fist of Cilantro

20 Grapes

6 Strawberries

8 Blackberries

1/4 inch Ginger Root (rhizome)

Pink Pump it Up Juice

3 Pink Lady Apples

8 large Strawberries

½ cup Red Raspberries

Morning Sunshine Juice

2 Carrots

20 Red and 20 Black seedless Grapes

½ inch Ginger root (rhizome)

6 Strawberries

1 red Apple

1 green Apple

4 leaves of Kale

1 Cucumber

Tropical Digestive-Booster Juice

½ Cantaloupe flesh

¼ Papaya flesh

½ Pineapple

<u>Energy Juice</u>

4 leaves of Kale

2 fist size bunches of Spinach

2 Celery stalks

¼ inch of Ginger root (rhizome)

20 Black seedless & 20 Red seedless Grapes

4 Strawberries

Fist size bunch of parsley

Fist size bunch of cilantro

1 cucumber

1 Green Apple and 1 Red Apple

¼ Pineapple

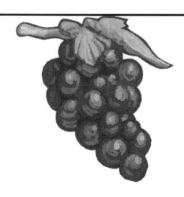

Jammin' Juice

15-20 Blueberries

2 red Apples

5 leaves Purple Cabbage

4 leaves of Kale

1 Cucumber

1 fist of Cilantro

Cit-Rush Juice

3 large Oranges (peeled)

2 large Limes (peeled)

2 large Lemons (peeled)

½ large Grapefruit (peeled)

<u>Midday and Afternoon Sustainability Juice</u>

4 leaves of Kale

2 fist of Spinach

1 Cucumber

½ inch Ginger root rhizome

1 Red Apple

1 Green Apple

20 Red and 20 Black seedless Grapes,

6 Strawberries

1 fist of Parsley

1 fist of Cilantro

1 Carrot

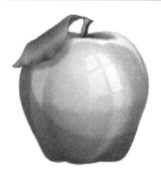

Cherry–licious!

20 pitted Cherries

4 Strawberries

3 Pears

1 apple

Paradise Juice

1 small bunch of red or black seedless grapes

½ pineapple

1 mango (skin and seed removed)

2 oranges

1 lime

1 lemon

Triple Grape Juice

1 small bunch of red seedless grapes

1 small bunch of green seedless grapes

1 small bunch of black seedless grapes

2 apples

Skin Refresher Juice

½ seedless Watermelon (juice flesh and rind)

1 large Cucumber

1 fist of parsley

1 fist of cilantro

2 apples

Strawberry Lime Juice

12 large Strawberries

4 large Limes (skin removed)

Tutti-Fruity Juice

3 whole kiwis (skin on)

2 Oranges (skin removed)

1 small bunch of seedless Green or Black Grapes

10 large Strawberries

Red Romance Juice

½ seedless or ¼ seeded watermelon (rind included)

2 Beet roots

3 red Apples

Small bunch red or black seedless Grapes

1 large Cucumber

2 Carrots

What's Up? Juice

5 Carrots

4 Celery stalks

2 large Apples

4 leaves of Romaine or Butter Lettuce

2 leaves of Cabbage

1 fist of Cilantro

Recovery Juice

6 leaves of Kale

2 fist size bunches of Spinach

4 Oranges (skin removed)

2 Apples

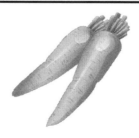

Kid's Favorite Juice

4 Apples

1 large Cucumber

2 Oranges (no skin)

¼ Pineapple

Coco Power Juice

Juice or Milk from one Coconut

8 large Strawberries

1 large Mango (skin and seed removed)

½ Pineapple

Berry Limeade Juice

4 Apples

1 Lime (skin removed)

8-10 Large Strawberries

Sunny Day Juice

2 Oranges (skin removed)

1 small Lime (skin removed)

¼ inch of Ginger root (rhizome)

2 red Apples

½ large Cucumber

Decision Making Juice

1 cup Blueberries

1 cup Blackberries

1 ½ cup pitted Cherries

4 leaves of Kale

1 small bunch of Spinach

2 Broccoli Florets with long stems

1 large Cucumber

1 large Apple

1 Lime (skin removed)

Stellar Stomach Buster Juice

2 red Apples

2 leaves Purple Cabbage

4 leaves of Kale

1 Cucumber

1 small bunch of Spinach

Clarity and Motion Juice

4 Carrots

½ inch of Ginger root (rhizome)

2 Lemons (skin removed)

Fist size bunch of parsley

3 Apples

Lett-us Juice

5 Lettuce leave (Romaine or your choice)

4 leaves of Kale

1 Cucumber

1 Apple

1 Orange

3 stalks of Celery

Bell-a Juice

1 Green Bell Pepper (seeds removed)

1 Red Bell Pepper (seeds removed)

2 fist size bunches of Spinach

3 Celery stalks

8 Strawberries

4 Apples

½ large Cucumber

Swamp Juice

2 Carrots

3 Red Apples

5 leaves Purple Cabbage

4 leaves of Kale

3 leaves of Collard Greens

1 large Cucumber

Easy-Joint Juice

6 Asparagus stalks

Fist size bunch of Parsley

Fist size bunch of Cilantro

1 large Cucumber

1 Green Apple and 1 Red Apple

2 stalks of Celery

1 large Broccoli Floret

2 Carrots

Juke Joint Juice

1 clove of Garlic

2 Roma Tomatoes

4 Carrots

1 Vidalia Onion

1 Cucumber

1 fist of Cilantro

Out Too Late Last Night Juice

4 Roma Tomatoes

4 Celery stalks

¼ of Ginger root (rhizome)

1 Lemon (skin removed)

Fist size bunch of parsley

1 Red Pepper (seeds removed)

1 Cucumber

Germ-Away Juice

6 Carrots

1 inch of Ginger root (rhizome)

1 Apple

Clarity Juice

2 large Cucumbers

Fist size bunch of Parsley

Fist size bunch of Cilantro

3 Green Apples

South of the Border Juice

2 red Apples

2 Limes (skin removed)

1 Jalapeno pepper

1 Cucumber

1 fist of Cilantro

This Ain't Kansas Juice

1 cup of peeled Jicama

2 Carrots

1 Green Apple and 1 Red Apple

¼ inch Ginger Root (rhizome)

Viva la Jugo! Juice

1 cup Cactus leaves (thorns removed & chopped)

2 Pears

2 Apples

4 leaves of Kale

1 Cucumber

1 fist of Cilantro

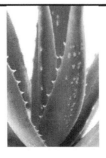

For the Long Haul Juice

4 leaves of Kale

2 fist size bunches of Spinach

20 Black seedless & 20 Red seedless Grapes

1 cucumber

1 Green Apple

1 Red Apple

Traveler's Delight Juice

4 red Apples

1 Cucumber

1 fist of Cilantro

Water-Bearer's Juice

Juice or Milk from 1 Coconut

1 Pomegranate (skin removed)

1 cup of Cherries (pits removed)

Aloe-Ha Juice

4 long Aloe Vera Stems

1 Pomegranate (skin removed)

1 large Cucumber

You Won't Forget this Juice

1 Grapefruit (skin removed)

1 fist size bunches of Spinach

4 leaves of Kale

¼ of Ginger root (rhizome)

Fist size bunch of parsley

Fist size bunch of cilantro

1 large Cucumber

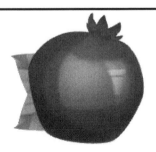

Springtime Juice

4 Apples

2 Pears

1 Peach

1 Plum

1 large Cucumber

Peaches N Cream Juice

4 Peaches

1 cup of fresh Coconut Milk

1 Mango (pit removed)

By the Beach Juice

1 Mango Pit removed

10 -12 Strawberries

3 Oranges

Wait a Minute! Juice

½ small seedless Watermelon

4 Tomatoes

2 Limes (skin removed)

2 Celery stalks

Good for the Blood Juice

5 leaves Purple Cabbage

2 Lemons (skin removed)

1 Cucumber

3 Pears

2 Apples

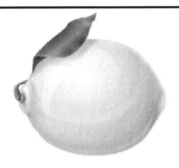

I Can Feel it in my Bones! Juice

2 fist size bunches of Spinach

¼ of Ginger root (rhizome)

Fist size bunch of parsley

1 Large cucumber

3 Apples

5 leaves of Red Cabbage

Dance Party Juice

4 red Apples

8 – 10 Strawberries

1 Lime (skin removed)

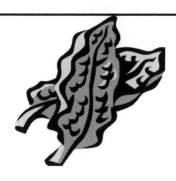

Like a Kid Again! Juice

4 leaves of Kale

2 fist size bunches of Spinach

2 leaves of Collard Greens

¼ of Ginger root (rhizome)

4 Oranges (skin removed)

Fist size bunch of parsley

1 Large Cucumber

2 Apples

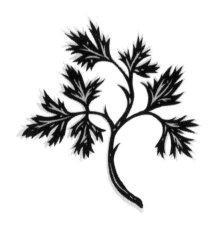

JUICE FOR THE ADVENTUROUS ONLY!!

Try these recipes if you can get your hands on these fruit during your travels!!

Exotica Juice

½ cup of Guarana berries

1 Guava - Goiaba

½ Brazilian Pineapple - Abacaxi

2 Acerola fruits

Brazil's Best Juice

2 Guavas - Goiaba

1 cup of Pitanga fruit

Like a Cherry Juice

2 cups of Pitanga fruit

2 cups of fresh Coconut Water

½ Brazilian Pineapple – Abacaxi

Fresh from the Feira! Juice

1 cup of Jabuticabas

½ Brazilian Pineapple – Abacaxi

Persimmons Perhaps?

4 Persimmons – Caqui fruit

1 Passion Fruit

1 Starfruit – Carambola

Summary

My tips for juicing recipes are as follows...start by following juice recipe directions as listed and adjust them to YOUR flavor!! I would also make notes directly in this book regarding changes that you made. That way you will not have to waste time trying to figure out your magic formula the next time you juice!!

It is also wise to make a shopping list of what you want to juice!

Here is a beginners shopping list:
1) 2-3 Heads of Kale

2) 2-3 bunches of Cilantro

3) 2-3 bunches of Parsley

4) 3-4 bunches of Spinach Leaves

5) 1-2 lbs of seedless Grapes (Black preferred, if

    available)

6) Large Ginger Root

7) Cucumbers (1 large per day or 2-3 small per day),

8) 6-8 lbs of red and/or green apples – I get both!

9) 2 Bunches of Carrots

7 Freshness – What to Buy? How to Store?

At the end of Chapter 6, I gave you a beginner's shopping list. Many of you already know how to select fruits and vegetables, but even seasoned produce shoppers love to hear tips on how to choose the best fruits and vegetables. But then when you get them home are we storing them appropriately? How many of us have thrown out wasted food, because we unintentionally accelerated the spoiling process? Well, this chapter is for you and you may become the produce connoisseur of your friends and family once you start sharing your tips!

The Organic Option!

While it would be my preference that all produce be grown organically, many countries and the vast majority of produce grown around the world does use some type of chemical pesticide, herbicide, etc. in order to increase yield. Unfortunately, chemical toxicants applied to crops are not the only issue. Now, genetically modified seeds are used in many crops around the world. Genetically modified organisms (GMOs) or genetically modified crops (GMCs) the plant's DNA – deoxyribonucleic acid is changed through genetic engineering to introduce a trait that is not found naturally. These changes can include resistance to certain diseases, faster and/or larger growth, resistance to chemicals, and production of a certain nutrient, resistance to weather or environmental conditions or the production of a pharmaceutical agent. Genetic modification by genetic engineering is completely different from selective breeding, in which the farmer may choose to save seeds and/or combined them with other plant varieties from certain naturally grown plants. Genetic engineering is very precise. In the short-term, there appears to be no health effects from consumption of GMOs or GMCs. You generally will not notice symptoms – unless you pay close attention to your body. But even those highly in tune with their body will find it difficult to notice immediate health changes by consuming these products. While the FDA, has stated that GMOs and GMCs are safe, long-term effects are unknown. Research is emerging showing adverse health effects in multiple animal species. While the debate rages on, I personally recommend organically produce and if organic is not available, local produce is the next best choice.

How to Pick them!!!

Many people know to avoid produce with bruises and blemishes and visible bugs. Some of us may need to d o a better job in avoiding those pests actively munching on our food! The following are some great tips to help you pick!

Check the sticker!!

- Produce grown with the use of pesticides and/or herbicides have a sticker or label with a 4 digit code usually starting with the number "4"

- Organic produce have a sticker or label that is a five digit code that usually starts with a "9" or "6"

Check the between the Cracks!!

- Look in between the leaves of lettuces, cabbages and greens. This way you can determine whether or not you can wash them out or if they have fully taken over!!

- Check in between the florets of broccoli and cauliflower. These are areas where insects can and will hide out and munch away!

Look for Sheen and Color!!

- Bright colors usually translate into tastier flavors and fresh micronutrients

- Look for a sheen, avoid dull produce. This indicates that it may be sitting longer. While they are still edible, this is not the freshest pick.

Weighty Issues!

- When picking up multiple pieces of the same type of produce choose the ones that appear heavier as this is also a freshness indicator

- Lighter produce may be older, drier and contaminated by pests

- This tip is most useful for fruits, but also can apply to some vegetables

Aroma…it smells so good!

- Ripe fruits and vegetables have a discernable scent!

- No scent indicates that the produce is not ripe

- Avoid produce that smells like the container that it was stored in

- Breathe in near where the stem was on the fruit or vegetable – here is where you can get a great indication of scent

Firmness!

- Your selection should be juicy – not too soft, not hard, but firm to the touch.

- You are looking for crispness in leafy vegetables.

- Pick up soft fruits gently and you will be able to feel whether or not they are firm.

- Figs and Hachiya persimmons are not firm – this tip does not apply to these fruits

Washing!

- Ensure that you are effectively washing your produce as soon as you bring them home

- Use a water and vinegar mix –

- You can use a 3 parts water to 1 part white vinegar (3:1) in a spray bottle – Spray produce and wash off thoroughly

- Produce Soak – I prefer a 4 parts water to 1 part white vinegar (4:1) soak of all produce for 20 minutes – Wash off thoroughly – note the dirt collected at bottom of bowl

- White vinegar can remove up to 98% of bacteria and will remove pesticide residues

- Use a vegetable scrub brush when washing off produce

- Never use bleach, soap or detergent to wash produce

Ethylene Gas & Spoilage

- As many fruits and vegetables proceed through the ripening process, they release ethylene gas

- Ethylene gas will make produce soften, become discolored or mealy (granular-like texture)

- Avoid mixing ethylene producing produce with ethylene sensitive produce

- Store ethylene producing produce in a separate drawer from ethylene sensitive produce

- Use paper, ethylene-removing or perforated storage bags for refrigeration/cold storage

Ethylene Producing Produce

- Apricot
- Avocado
- Banana
- Cantaloupe
- Honeydew melon
- Kiwi
- Mango
- Nectarine
- Papaya
- Peach
- Pear
- Plums
- Tomato

Ethylene Sensitive Produce

- Apples
- Asparagus
- Broccoli
- Carrots
- Cucumbers
- Eggplants
- Green beans
- Lettuce and other greens

- Potatoes
- Summer squash
- Watermelons

Where to Store Produce!

- Often times we may spend a lot of time choosing and cleaning our produce only to stick them all into cold storage
- Some produce should be stored at room temperature to ensure proper ripening and best quality flavor and nutrition
- Certain produce should be stored in cold storage to extend their edible life
- Some produce should be stored at room temperature to ripen, then transferred into storage to extend their edible life (after ripening store and use within 1-3 days)
- You can use a paper bag to accelerate ripening of produce that is ripened at room temperature and then transferred into cold storage

Whew!! So where do I store?? The following chart will help!!

Storage Chart! Keep this Handy!

Room Temperature Storage	Room temperature ripening then Refrigerator Storage	Refrigerator Cold Storage
Apple (for 7 days or less)	Avocado	Apple (longer than 7 days)
Banana	Kiwi	Apricot
Basil (in water)	Nectarine	Asian Pear
Citrus Fruits	Peach	Artichoke
Cucumber	Pear	Asparagus
Eggplant	Plum	Beet (cut off 2in above crown)
Garlic	Pluot/Plumcots	Berries
Ginger		Broccoli
Jicama		Brussel Sprout
Mango		Cabbage
Melons		Carrot

Room Temperature Storage	Room temperature ripening then Refrigerator Storage	Refrigerator Cold Storage
Papaya		Cauliflower
Peppers		Celery
Persimmons		Cherries
Pineapple		Coconut
Plantain		Endive
Pomegranate		Figs
Potatoes		Grapes
Pumpkin		Green Beans
Sweet Potato		Green Onions
Tomato		Herbs (except Basil)
Winter Squash		Leafy Vegetables
		Leeks

Room Temperature Storage	Room temperature ripening then Refrigerator Storage	Refrigerator Cold Storage
		Lettuce
		Mushrooms
		Peas
		Radish
		Spinach
		Sprouts
		Summer Squash
		Sweet Corn
		Zucchini

- Cucumber, Eggplant and Peppers can be stored in the refrigerator for 1-3 days, then used quickly. Store Away from Direct Sunlight

- Store Garlic, Onions, Potatoes, Sweet Potatoes in well ventilated area away from sunlight

- Store all CUT fruits and vegetables in refrigerator

- Store Kale, Lettuces and Leafy Greens in an aerated plastic bag lined with a paper towel

- Produce should be stored in their own aerated or ethylene removing storage bags

- Kiwis should be ripened in a warm, humid place

- Berries should be refrigerated uncovered or in an aerated storage container

Peak Season Guide!!!

Use the following guide to pick your produce at the best time of year!!

Name of Fruit	In Season
Apple	September – May
Apricot	June – July
Avocado	All Year

Name of Fruit	In Season
Banana	All Year
Berries – Blueberry	June – August
Berries – Cranberry	September – December & March – July
Berries – Strawberry	June – August
Cherry	May - June
Coconut	September – March
Figs	July – September
Grapefruit	October – June
Grapes	June – December
Kiwi	June – August
Lemon	All Year
Lime	May – October
Mango	April – August
Melons – Cantaloupe	May – September
Melons – Casabas	July – October
Melons – Crenshaws	July – October
Melons – Honeydews	February – October
Melons – Persians	July – October

Name of Fruit	In Season
Melons – Watermelon	May – October
Nectarine	June – September
Orange	November – June
Peach	June – September
Papaya	All Year
Pear	August – May
Persimmons	October – January
Pineapple	February – August
Plum	June – September
Pomegranate	September – November
Tangerines	November – January
Tangelos	January – October
Name of Vegetable	**In Season**
Artichoke	March – May
Asparagus	March – June
Beans – Green	April – October
Beans – Limas	April – August
Beans – Wax	April – October
Beet	June – October

Name of Vegetable	In Season
Broccoli	October – May
Brussel Sprouts	October – November
Cabbage	All Year
Cauliflower	September – November
Celery	All Year
Corn	May – September
Cucumbers	May – August
Eggplant	August – September
Endive (Belgian)	October - May
Kale	Mid-Summer – December
Lettuce	All Year
Mushrooms	November – April
Okra	May – September
Onions	All Year
Parsnips	October – April
Peas (Green)	April – July
Peppers	All Year
Potato – White	All Year
Potato – Sweet	September – December

Name of Vegetable	In Season
Radish	May – July
Spinach	March – May
Squash – Summer	June – August
Squash – Winter	September – November
Tomato	May – August
Turnips	Rutabagas
Watercress	May – November
Name of Herb	**In Season**
Basil	February – September
Chamomile	February – September
Chives	All Year
Cilantro	All Year
Dill	February – September
Mint	All Year
Oregano	February – September
Parsley	All Year
Rosemary	All Year
Sage	February – September
Stevia	February – September

Name of Herb	In Season
Sweet Marjoram	February – September
Tarragon	February – September
Thyme	February – September

Summary

While this chapter does not cover all fruits and vegetables, you will likely be able to better identify exotic fruits at their freshest once you start using the tips from this chapter!

8 Documenting my Juice Feast Journey on Social Media!

When I decided to start juicing years ago, I must admit it was because I simply did not like eating a lot of fruits and vegetables on a daily basis and I wanted to be able to incorporate more plant based items in my diet. Juicing was great, but it took me a while to understand what I needed to juice to gain the maximum benefit. Over the years, I realized how wonderful incorporating juicing was into my diet, but I did not juice on a daily basis. Despite the fact that my body appeared to be responding well to the juice, I kept falling back into my traditional mostly cooked, animal protein based diet.

Now, I am still not a vegan or vegetarian, but I have learned that by significantly reducing my intake of animal based meals and increasing the number of plant-based meals, that I have increased energy, better digestion and a better mood and outlook. While everyone will respond differently to a nutritional plan – simply due to our unique genetic makeup, we all require the same types of macronutrients (protein, carbohydrates and fats) and micronutrients (vitamins and minerals). We require a much smaller amount of micronutrients, hence the "micro" prefix. Deficiency, especially in micronutrients leads to disease. So how did I get to a 30 day straight juice feast? I decided to try going on a 100% raw juice feast. Initially, I thought I would try to juice for a few days, 3 at most, but 3 turned into 30 and I wanted to share my juice feast with others on social media! I received so many e-mails and messages of support from my "Dr Noreen" family! And many of them were inspired to juice with great results! Here are some of my social media posts.

Days 1-3

The first two days were the most challenging. My juice was filling and I was not hungry, but boy was it hard to smell my family's food. As a matter of fact, I told them to fend for themselves and I would go into the other room to avoid the aromas.

"Hi everyone!! Just want to give you an update on what I have been up to. I finally started my juice feast!! I am consuming fresh juice and water! So last night (day 3) I went to bed at 3 am and woke up at 6:30 a.m. refreshed. I forced myself to lay there another 30 min and then I got up and started cleaning up! Did I mention that I went out last night (drank water with twist of fresh lime juice)? And for those wondering what time my last juice was consumed yesterday,

I had 24 oz of my green juice at 8 pm. The energy that I have is great! I must admit day 1 and 2 were tough but I'm good today....and I turned down the brisket that my husband just brought home!

I have not set a firm number of days that I will juice feast. I am basically taking it day by day, but at this point I will at least juice for 7 days! I will keep you posted and let me know if you have any questions! I did transition from eating raw meals and raw juice for several days before I went to straight juice feasting!

Oh, and I have lost 5 lbs in 4 days!

Here is my beginner's juice recipe!

<u>Starter Juice:</u>

2 medium apples

2-3 medium carrots

1 cucumber

4 large strawberries

Handful of seedless grapes (red, white or both)

1/4 inch ginger root (rhizome)

Juice and enjoy! I recommend juicing the ginger halfway through the juicing process! Don't forget to #share this with others!!"

Day 5

Today's juice update! So I stepped on the scale this morning and noticed that I am now missing 8 lbs. Yes! I was a little tired because I was working on the 3.5 hrs from Saturday night (night 3) and 5 hrs from last night (night 4 - long story but basically had too much energy to go to sleep). Today's breakfast and lunch juice:

Lovely Green Juice:

4 leaves of kale

2 fist-size bunches of spinach

1 cucumber

4 small apples

Fist size bunch of parsley,

Fist size bunch of cilantro,

20 grapes,

6 strawberries,

8 blackberries

and 1/4 inch ginger root (rhizome).

Very tasty! Drank lots of water and did some light exercise (squats and push-ups). So far I'm quite pleased, but I will be trying to get to bed earlier as sleep is critical to good health! #share my juice journey with your friends! And my inbox has been buzzing...keep the questions coming!"

Day 6

"Feeling really good! I think that I can do this for a little longer! I must admit I just smelled some really good food cooking (so I did this Jedi mind trick and pretended that I just ate what I was smelling...and it worked)! And....drum-roll please......I lost another 3 lbs! 11 lbs down in 6 days and I can certainly feel it in my clothes. Now, I am waiting on these arms to start shrinking too! I did 50 modified push-ups, 60 squats, arm and waist exercises!

Today's Power juice:

20 red seedless grapes,

4 leaves of kale,

1 inch ginger root (rhizome)

2 fist size bunches of spinach,

Fist size bunch of cilantro,

Fist size bunch parsley,

2 carrots,

1 cucumber

I used a lot of ginger and the juice was nice and spicy"

Day 7

"Thirteen lbs lost!!!

Today's Energy juice:

4 leaves of kale,

2 fist size bunches of spinach,

2 celery stalks,

¼ of ginger (rhizome),

20 black grapes,

20 red grapes,

4 strawberries,

Fist size bunch of parsley,

Fist size bunch of cilantro,

1 cucumber,

1 green apple

1 red apple and

¼ pineapple.

I have never been a fan of the taste of celery (in my juice), but I wanted to try again. Conclusion: still not a fan as the flavor is overpowering; so I will reduce the quantity in the future. Last night I made a fruit juice!

Evening Energy Fruit juice:

20 red and 20 black grapes,

1 green apple,

½ cucumber,

¼ ginger and

6 strawberries

It was amazing! Very refreshing and it made me feel better as I smelled my husband's BBQ chicken. So I'm not sure how many more days that I will juice feast..."

Day 8

"Day 8!! Total of 15 lbs lost!!! 2 more pounds missing from my body!! Got back into my size 4! Feeling good (and maybe a little vain...but it's always nice to get into the dress that you REALLY want to wear). I have been much busier than usual this week and I have not had a problem with energy! My skin feels a lot softer, which is very nice. I have had no adverse reactions or symptoms. I would like to keep going at least a few more days...we will see!"

Today's Morning Sunshine juice:

2 carrots,

20 red and 20 black grapes,

½ inch ginger,

6 strawberries,

1 red apple

1 green apple

4 leaves of kale

1 cucumber

<u>Midday and Afternoon Sustainability juice</u>:

4 leaves of kale,

2 fist size bunches of spinach,

1 cucumber,

½ inch ginger,

1 red and

1 green apple,

20 red and 20 black grapes,

6 strawberries,

1 fist size bunch of parsley,

1 fist size bunch of cilantro, and

1 carrot.

<u>Day 9</u>

"It's Day 9 of my juice feasting!!! Thanks to everyone that has enquired about taking a juicing journey of their own!! As a toxicologist, I know how important it is to support your body's detoxification system. Deciding to "eat" juice instead of food sounds crazy (because I love to chew), but it makes so much sense!! My digestive system needed a good rest from digesting animal protein and cooked foods.

I will tell you that yesterday and today I felt the urge to eat (several times). I had not felt the urge to eat since the first 2 days and I had to figure out why!! I believe that it may be due to the carrot that I have put in my juice yesterday and today. Carrots are high in sugar and even though I am not a diabetic, I try to limit high glycemic foods as much as possible. Glycemic cycling is detrimental to your body and can cause you to feel hungry. So I am going to stop the carrot and see if that makes a difference.

So Sunday is Mother's Day and I have not decided whether I should stop my juice feasting or not. Since I am taking this day by day, I will decide for sure tomorrow. What do you guys think??

By the way, I lost one more pound (16 lbs) total!! Cheering for myself!!!"

Lovely Green Juice:

4 leaves of kale

2 fist-size bunches of spinach

1 cucumber

4 small apples

Fist size bunch of parsley,

Fist size bunch of cilantro,

20 grapes,

6 strawberries,

8 blackberries

and 1/4 inch ginger root (rhizome).

Day 10

"Today is Day 10!!!! I lost another pound!!! 17 lbs total in 10 days!

If anyone wants to go shopping today for your juicing produce here are the basics that I recommend:

Dr. Noreen's Juice-Feasting Shopping List:
1) 2-3 bunches of kale,

2) 2-3 bunches of cilantro,

3) 2-3 bunches of parsley,

4) 3-4 bunches of spinach,

5) 1-2 lbs of seedless grapes,

6) Large ginger root,

7) Cucumbers (1 large per day or 2-3 small per day),

8) 6-8 lbs of red and or green apples)!

Come juice with me! And I have decided (as my husband is grilling chicken) that I am going to keep going!!! No break for Mother's Day!"

Day 12

"Day 12!! And some of you have decided to join me on a juice feast! I'm so proud of you! I won't call out your names until you tell me it's ok. And keep me posted on your daily journey! And take measurements so that young can document the inches lost! I have lost a total of 18 lbs!!! I made a special Mother's Day juice yesterday!

Today's juice: Dr Noreen's green juice!"

Dr. Noreen's Green Juice:

4 leaves of Kale,

½ inch ginger,

1 large cucumber,

1 fist size bunch of cilantro,

1 fist size bunch of parsley,

4 apples!

Day 13

"Day 13 of my Juice Feast! I am so excited to say that I am missing 19 lbs (8.6 kgs)! So I am hoping that I can make it at least 20 lbs by tomorrow (2 weeks)!! WOO-HOO I AM SO EXCITED!!"

Dr. Noreen's Green Juice (morning):

4 leaves of Kale,

½ inch ginger,

1 large cucumber,

1 fist size bunch of cilantro,

1 fist size bunch of parsley,

1 bunch of spinach

4 apples!

Lovely Green Juice (afternoon and evening):

4 leaves of kale

2 fist-size bunches of spinach

1 cucumber

4 small red or green apples

Fist size bunch of parsley,

Fist size bunch of cilantro,

20 grapes,

6 strawberries,

8 blackberries

and 1/4 inch ginger root (rhizome).

Day 14

"Day 14! 2 weeks! Woo-hoo! When I started my juice feast I did not know how long I would be able to sustain this, but here I am 2 weeks later feeling awesome! And I am now missing 20 lbs! I have heard that weight loss will slow and then pick up as you continue to juice. I must admit that while I did not start for weight loss, I could not be more pleased!

Today's juice: Lovely Green Juice

<u>Lovely Green Juice</u>:

4 leaves of kale

2 fist-size bunches of spinach

1 cucumber

4 small red or green apples

Fist size bunch of parsley,

Fist size bunch of cilantro,

20 seedless grapes (white, red or black),

6 strawberries,

8 blackberries

and 1/4 inch ginger root (rhizome).

Afternoon juice snack -

<u>Sweet Snack Juice</u>:

2 small oranges,

3 large strawberries,

1 red apple!

(Tasted like candy!)

So excited for all of you that have inboxes me your e-mail address so that you can start your own juice feast!"

<u>Day 16</u>

"Woo-hoo y'all! Day 16, feeling great! 21 lbs missing! I am so amazed at how much better my skin feels! Not that my skin was rough before, but it is much better now! Even my feet are softer, which is the area that gives many of us problems! So today I juiced purple cabbage for the first time. It has a very mild earthy taste. I will use it again in the future. If you try start with 1-2 leaves, I juiced 5 ... A few too many! My energy levels are very good and I have noticed that I need to up my water intake as well. My body wants more!

<u>Jammin' Juice recipe</u>:

15-20 blueberries,

2 red apples,

5 leaves purple cabbage,

4 leaves of kale,

1 cucumber,

1 fist size bunch of cilantro.

A less complicated juice alternative (for beginners):

<u>Apple-berry Refresher</u>:

2 apples

1 cucumber

20 blueberries

My daughter told me that she is tired of me juicing because I can't eat with her. (Awwww) When I explained how much better I feel she told me to keep going!

I am so excited that many of you have started your transition phase and are eating your raw meals and raw juicing! Shout out to [*Name Removed*] who said she had one of the best tasting meals (raw or cooked) when she had her raw meal today! I love that so many of you are open to improving your health and joining me on a juice feast! Please continue to update me and share my statuses with your friends and family. So many people are looking for a change and a support system. This page has many answers to several questions that have been asked! Please encourage them to like my page so that they can receive my status updates too!

My juice guide will be published soon! Thank you all and I appreciate all of the great comments and support that you give to me!"

Day 20

"It's DAY 20!!!! I cannot believe how wonderful this nutrition change has been for me! As of today, I feel wonderful, my skin looks great (and feels great), I have great energy and I have "divorced" 23 POUNDS from my body!!! My husband loves it and has been very encouraging!

So I have gotten so many questions about protein & carbohydrates and the difference between juicing and blending. So, I am addressing this for you now.

There are proteins and carbohydrates in fruits and vegetables (look it up and verify)! So, when you juice an array of protein and carbohydrate containing vegetables, you are not deficient.

Now if you don't juice a wide variety of fruits and vegetables you can become deficient, so get that wide variety of colors and flavors!! I love being able to consume so many fruits and vegetables in a nice easy glass of juice!! I could never physically eat this many fruits and veggies in a day!

We have been taught that animal proteins are the best and this is because they contain 20 of the 20 amino acids that we need for all of our biochemical processes throughout the body. We as human produce 10 of our 20 amino acids so we are deficient in the other 10, which we obtain from our diet. Vegetables contain some but not all of the 20 amino acids (and that is why they are incomplete proteins). When you eat or juice a wide variety of plant based proteins, you get all of the amino acids that you require! So any of the nay-sayers that tell you that you are deficient because you juice or consume all plant based meals are WRONG. And you cannot overdo it with plant based proteins! Get enough calories and your body will be happy! Plus with the right juicer you can even juice nuts!

Unfortunately, consuming too much animal protein, can be very destructive and has been shown to cause disease and/or damage to the kidneys, liver and colon (major detoxification organs).

LET ME BE CLEAR - I AM NOT A VEGAN OR VEGETARIAN! [*But if I was, I would be a proud one!*] I love the taste of animal proteins, but I do not love the havoc that they wreak on my body! I have not felt this good in years! I am not bloated after I eat certain foods (a sure fire signal that your body is rejecting or reacting adversely to what you eat). I do miss chewing every once in a while, but that will come in time! I have been chewing for decades so a few weeks off are due! And, I will be a fully raw vegan (raw plant based) diet once I stop juicing, then I will transition to a vegan (all plant based, some cooked) diet, then vegetarian (some animal proteins such as eggs allowed) and then pescetarian (sea-based proteins like fish). Eventually, I will eat land-based animal proteins, but this will be severely restricted. I cannot go back to eating animal proteins daily and ignoring my body's "reject" symptoms. This is my plan for now and I will let you know if I make any adjustments!

EXERCISE- So there really should be no issue continuing any workout plan that you are on. However, it is not wise to start a new workout plan as you adjust to a new diet. Allow your body time to acclimate to your nutrition before starting any new workout plan. (Consult your physician)

I have been doing the squat challenge and various callisthenic exercises. No joint pains or muscle aches to report.

THE DIFFERENCE BETWEEN JUICING & BLENDING:

First, I recommend a low speed masticating juicer.

Juicing releases more micronutrients from the plant cell wall than blending will. Blending does not separate these essential micronutrients from the plant fiber. This is why you should not fall for the marketing that says blenders can juice. Blenders can kill many of the beneficial micronutrients by heating and killing them with high power motors. ANY

PRODUCT THAT HAS THE WORD MIXER OR BLENDER IN THE TITLE IS NOT A JUICER!! I cannot stress this enough. So while you think it's much better to drink the fiber soup that your blender calls juice, you are NOT getting the best juice possible.

Centrifugal juicers are good too (I used one for years) but they are not nearly as good as the low speed masticating juicer. You lose a lot of your good juice in the pulp in a centrifugal juicer. The low speed masticating juicer puts out the driest pulp and you can always run your juice through a hand strainer if you don't want any bits or fiber.

My advice is not meant to treat, cure or diagnose any medical conditions that you may have. Always consult a physician before making a change in your nutrition and exercise (which means you should have consulted your physician before you started hitting up those fast food joints years ago)! If you are on medications, make certain that they are not contraindicated with certain plant based foods

Why do people ask so many questions about something that is good for you, but it takes a news report before they find out that much of their burger is made from ammonia treated beef throwaways? Are you asking all those questions about your processed food? Don't be a nutrition hypocrite!

Please share this post with your family and friends them and ask them to like my page!! And use food to help fight the toxic effects of environmental exposure!

Day 22

"Good morning!!! Its day 22 and I am 25 lbs lighter! Today's juice recipe:

Purple Power Juice:
2 leaves of Swiss chard,
green grapes,
2 leaves purple kale,
1 cucumber,
1 orange,
4 strawberries,
1 pear,
1 kiwi,
2 red and 2 green apples,
1 fist size bunch of spinach,
1 fist size bunch cilantro,
20 blueberries

Have a wonderful day!"

Day 25

"Day 25!! T minus 5 days!! I have decided to transition off of my juice feast after 30 days!! So Saturday, I will have my first meal!!
I have made great juices this week and I have cooked a LOT this weekend! This is because I am trying to prepare meals for next week for my family. But I also tried something TOTALLY NEW! I made vegetarian black bean burgers from

scratch! They looked and smelled wonderful...but of course I could not sample! So instead, I fed them to my daughter, aunt and 2 uncles! They all thought that that their "burgers" were very good! YAY! I am excited because they are all meat eaters. So I have made several patties in advance and I will eat them once I start incorporating vegetarian meals back in. I know that strict vegans and vegetarians frown on making fake "meat" meals, but I think that these options are excellent, especially if you are trying to transition away from eating meat. Here is my "fave" new morning juice!"

SWEET CANDY JUICE:

2 oranges,

2 apples,

6 - 8 large strawberries

YUMMY! I can see now, that once I start allowing meat back into my diet, that I will be making most of my days vegetarian and limiting meat to 1-2 times per week. So WHY am I stopping at 30 days? Well, I have a wedding anniversary, birthday and vacations coming up in June! And my juice feasting has me ready to celebrate! I will continue to raw juice daily and I am so glad that I have been able to share this journey with you!"

Day 28

"Day 28!!! I am 26 lbs lighter and very happy with how I feel! Some of you have seen me in person and have pointed out how much smaller that I am.

By the way, I have noticed that my allergies are not getting to me! While others around me suffer. Grass pollen is one of my big issues - the counts were HIGH on Monday and Medium yesterday and today. This would normally be an issue, but I walked around outside with no problems!!! I am not 100% certain that this is due to my juicing - because I have not checked my blood biomarkers, but I do believe that my nutrition is making a difference! I hope this continues, because my seasonal allergies were really bothering me a few weeks ago! I am looking forward to eating an avocado on Saturday!! Weird? Maybe, but I am excited about my raw food transition! And yes, I will be eating more than an avocado on Saturday!!

Please keep your juice updates coming! Wins and setbacks! Setbacks are just a set up for a comeback! So keep on juicing! Even if you do not change anything else about your diet, it is a GREAT way to get a lot of plant based foods into your system quickly. And we can all use more greens (unless you are already a raw vegan)! Today, I had melon juice!"

<u>Tropical Digestive-Booster Juice</u>:

½ cantaloupe flesh

¼ papaya flesh

Very filling and great for the digestive system. LOVED IT!"

Day 30

"It is day 30!! My final juice feast day!!! I will have my final weigh in tomorrow morning. I lost another 1/2 lb yesterday! I have been planning my raw meals out and I even bought some vegetarian "cheese" substitute!

Today's Green Juice:

4 leaves of kale,

2 fist-size bunches of spinach,

1 fist size bunch of parsley,

20 black grapes,

3 apples,

2 oranges,

½ inch ginger,

6 strawberries

Day 31

(First eating day): "Hello everyone! Hope you are enjoying your weekend! So I weighed in this morning and logged a total of 27 lbs!! So what was my first bite of food? A medjool date! It was so good! Then I ate a bowl of raw oatmeal with, organic chia seeds, homemade almond milk, organic blueberries and raspberries and chopped medjool dates. It was very good! And later I made my guacamole! Yum! I noticed that my stomach has shrunk because I get full much faster than I did previously! I am very pleased about that!

Also I juiced half of a small seedless watermelon (rind included). Super delicious!!! I just whipped up my first batch of raw hummus for later on! I will let you know if this is a success or a mistake tomorrow. But the small taste test was promising! I also took a walk earlier today.

By the way, I made the almond milk by juicing my almonds (soaked raw almonds overnight and juiced with filtered water). Tastes so much better than store bought! I do love my masticating juicer because I could never do that or juice a watermelon in my old centrifugal juicer!"

Summary

So that was my social media journey through juicing! It is fun to have a support system. My social media fan page http://www.facebook.com/DoctorNoreen (please like) was just the support that I needed! I was really inspired to keep going, not just for my health, but to show others that they too can juice feast! I am not super-human and the internet is now filled with testimonies from people who have juiced 30, 60 even 90 days or more! I hope you noticed the Transitioning Phases, which I discussed in Chapter 4. I believe that this component is just one element that makes my juice guide different from all of the rest and will help set you up for success!

9 Beware of false Medical Cures and Promises tied to Fruits and Vegetables!

While I am all for using my consumption of fruits and vegetables as a means to meet my bodies needs in order to prevent the occurrence of disease and boost natural detoxification; I am not pleased when I see medical promises or cures tied to plant based foods (or man-made chemicals if it's not true). It is important to note that countless scientists and physicians work diligently to cure and prevent disease. However, ethical persons in the field of science and medicine, never promise more than they can deliver. Unfortunately, some people promoting health and wellness will over-promise and often under-deliver. They may be well intentioned, but they do not realize the countless people that they ultimately harm by not providing fact-based information.

I have seen and read juice books that promise cures for

acne, diabetes, cancer, you-name-it-disease-of-the-month, etc, etc. This is simply unethical and gives false hopes to some who have done too much damage for any natural or man-made cure to work. While research may support some amazing or even slight improvements to those suffering with disease by consuming plant based foods, they are not a cure all. Emerging research does provide us hope that one day, we can find the magic combination of plant based foods that will prevent any health related issue.

Unfortunately, no plant or vegetable, or combination thereof, is widely accepted as the cure to ANY disease. However, consumption of a plant based diet or adding more plant based foods or juices to your regular diet can and often improves many health conditions for people suffering from disease. It can even prevent the onset of disease. But we must remain aware that we all have a varied genetic makeup and we are constantly exposed to toxic chemicals in our environment. Therefore, despite our best efforts disease can still occur. But never despair! Instead, treat the one body that we have for this lifetime as best as we possibly can. And the best way to do that is to ensure that our bodies have the required amounts of macro and micronutrients.

Personally, I would have never bothered to write a book about juicing to support detoxification, if I had not reviewed loads of research and literature supporting health benefits of plant based foods – and seen and felt amazing improvements in my own life! And yes, dropping the weight felt good too! Now you are ready to pack in those micronutrients. Please do me a favor and let me know your amazing juicing stories and great juice recipes!!

The formula is easy! Now get to your juicers and make some NOISE!!!! The next chapter is all yours for you to track your juicing experiences!!

10 Tracking Your Progress!

This section is for you to write. Here you should write down how you feel, what you love or dislike! Your goals health and/or weight-wise! Or you can simply make notes! This is ALL about YOU!!

Tips:
- Take measurements first
- Write down current weight and goal weight (if you intend to gain or lose weight)
- Write down current energy levels and any symptoms or issues that you experience on a routine basis!
- Note any Medications

Name: _____

Date: _____ Weight: _____

Measurements: _____

Symptoms:_____

_____

GOALS:

_____

_____

_____

_____

_____

_____

_____

_____

_____

_____

_____

_____

_____

_____

_____

_____

COOL STUFF: CHANGES IN ENERGY, MOOD, ETC..

_____

_____

_____

_____

_____

_____

_____

_____

_____

_____

_____

_____

_____

_____

_____

_____

_____

_____

_____

_____

_____

_____

_____

_____

_____

_____

_____

_____

_____

_____

LIKES/DISLIKES ABOUT JUICING

MY OWN RECIPES:

_____

_____

_____

_____

_____

_____

_____

_____

_____

_____

_____

_____

_____

_____

NOTES FOR HEALTH CARE PROVIDER:

_____

_____

_____

_____

_____

_____

_____

_____

_____

_____

_____

_____

_____

_____

_____

BEFORE and AFTER PHOTOS

ABOUT THE AUTHOR

Noreen Khan-Mayberry, PhD was born in New York City, New York and grew up in Houston, Texas. Dr. Noreen, also known as "The Tox Doc", is a Toxicologist that specializes in environmental, space, food and nutritional toxicology. Her personal mission is to translate the language of science for non-scientists in order to educate and inform the public of critical issues that affect their health and quality of life. Dr. Noreen has been featured on television (as seen on CBS & Fox) talk radio (as heard on K-ABC) as a guest expert and she is an active public speaker that has spoken internationally. Her book "Talking Toxicology" is an essential guide that provides an easy to understand breakdown of the science of toxicology and how to recognize and reduce toxic exposures.

Dr. Noreen is serving as an editorial member of the Journal of Clinical Toxicology and The International Journal of Disaster Advances. Dr. Noreen has been with NASA* since 2004 and worked as the first female Space Toxicologist. She has authored a number of research articles in Space Toxicology, Environmental Toxicology and planetary dust toxicity. She has served as the lead author of the first chapter ever published on the specialty of Space Toxicology in an international toxicology textbook. She is a Fellow of the International Congress of Disaster Management and a member of the Society of Toxicology and the American College of Toxicology. She has been honored as a Woman as Global Leaders, 2013 Trailblazer Award for Science Technology Engineering and Math (STEM), 2013 & 2012 Award of Excellence from the Council of Inspector Generals on Integrity and Efficiency (CIGIE), 2010 Technology Rising Star among several other awards.

*The information and statements contained in this work are the professional opinion of the author and are not endorsed, sponsored or representative of the United States Federal government or any Federal Agency.

Made in the USA
Charleston, SC
01 October 2013